The Keto Diet Planner

The Total Keto Meal Diet Planning Guide

GW00382122

a result of the use of information contained within this document, including, but not limited to, —errors, omissions, or inaccuracies.

Table of Contents

Introduction

The ketogenic diet is simply a lifestyle change that includes the involvement of foods with low carbohydrates and high fat content. The diet is also well known as the low carb diet or the low carb, high fat diet.

When you eat a lot of carbohydrates, they often turn to sugar, triggering your body to produce large amounts of glucose and insulin. This can be a problem because glucose is actually one of the easiest molecules for your body to break down, meaning that your body is going to burn the glucose instead of the fat that is already stored in your body. When this happens, you can end up gaining weight.

This diet, the "keto diet," helps you lose weight by eliminating—or at least reducing—the effect that eating large amounts of carbohydrates causes. When you do not eat so many carbohydrates and eat more fat, your body will want to burn the fat for energy. During the times that you do not eat, your body will burn some of what is left over, as well. This will give you a boost in fat loss and weight management.

The diet is based on the process of ketosis, which is basically the process by which the body initiates when food intake is low. Ketosis is kind of like a defense mechanism when the body is hungry. We produce *ketones* that break down fat in the liver in response to what our body thinks is starvation. The whole point of the ketogenic diet is to force the body into this state of ketosis, speeding up the metabolism and burning fat all day long.

So why does this work so well?

Well, the body is "very adaptive to what you put into it" (ruled.me), meaning that when you pack it full of healthy fats—like almonds and avocado—and reduce your daily intake of carbohydrates, your body is going to start burning ketones as it's primary energy source right away.

In the following pages, you will learn that there are many benefits to this diet. You'll also learn which foods to avoid and which ones to embrace during your new lifestyle change. Recipes and a fully laid out diet plan that you can follow and love will be included as well!

Chapter One: The Essentials - Different Types of Ketogenic Diets

Even though the ketogenic diet is quite straightforward, you'll notice that there are modifications that can be made. In fact, there are three different types of ketogenic diets, those being the standard, targeted and cyclic ketogenic diets.

All three versions of the ketogenic diet follow the same idea. However, there is a slight different in each one. Here they are explained.

The Standard Ketogenic Diet

This is the ketogenic diet that has been explained earlier. The goal is to simply eat a smaller amount of carbohydrates. This causes the body to burn less sugars as the primary energy source, making your body burn fat instead. The diet requires a minimum if about "20-50 grams of carbs a day" (letodietapp.com) - as you can see, you should really restrict your carbohydrates.

Many people find that this is the best diet to go on when you are first getting used to the ketogenic idea. People find this one the best due to the tracking, scheduling, and training that you may encounter in the other two (you will see that momentarily). This is the easiest ketogenic diet to keep track of, therefor being the favorite amongst most beginners.

Even though there aren't any things to really plan, you do have to keep track of the amount of fat and carbohydrates that you are consuming. As we already know, you should always aim for high fat and low carbs.

Targeted Ketogenic Diet

This ketogenic diet is a little different than the other two. It is slightly more revolved around exercise and what you eat before your workout. When you are not working out, you will eat good foods, avoiding carbohydrates, like the standard ketogenic diet. The biggest—and only real—difference that you see in the targeted ketogenic diet is that before your workout you eat about 20 to 50 grams of carbohydrates.

Wait... What?

Yeah! You should eat extra carbs before you work out. Many people find that consuming their carbs about 30 to 60 minutes before a workout is the most effective way to go about this diet. It is important to know that post-workout meals are to be high in protein and carbohydrates as well as low in fat.

Usually, the ketogenic diet entails high fats and low carbs, but in this version of the diet it is only the opposite before a workout. The idea is to work off both fat and carbohydrates during a workout to achieve optimal weight loss and toning. Another important thing to note is to avoid foods high in fat for a while after your workout, as well. This is because fat after a workout has been proven to hinder some nutrient absorption and muscle recovery.

When on this type of ketogenic diet, it is also a good idea to do body weight and resistance training. This way, you will burn off as much fat as you possibly can, while gaining muscle and toning your body. Some of the best methods to tone and gain muscle are yoga, calisthenics and strength or resistance training. These methods engage certain muscle groups in the body, enabling you to target those places that you feel you need to improve on.

Cyclic Ketogenic Diet

Before I begin, I should let you fellow readers know that not everyone is able to keep track of this form of the ketogenic diet. The targeted and cyclic ketogenic diets are said to not be completely suitable for everyone. This is due to the planning and effort that often come along with them.

So, what is the third ketogenic diet?

The cyclic ketogenic diet involves carb cycling and carb back loading. This simply means that you will be choosing certain days where you will be following the standard ketogenic diet, while other days you will eat mostly carbs. This is what is known as "carb-loading." When you carb-load and when you decide to avoid carbs are completely up to you; it usually depends on your personal preference and your schedule.

When you are on the ketogenic part of the diet, it is recommended that you eat only about 50 grams of carbohydrates. We can compare this to the 450 to 600 grams of carbohydrates that you are encouraged to consume on the days that you are carb-loading. This diet is often used when people want to build excess amounts of muscle. These people often involve certain athletes like bodybuilders and people who regularly perform bodyweight exercises like calisthenics.

You should be aware of the disclaimer that should be given when you talk about the cyclic ketogenic diet: you may gain weight. If this diet is not used to build muscle and if the diet is not used or performed correctly, you could end up gaining weight instead of building muscle. So, make sure to talk to a personal trainer or doctor to find out the best way to build muscle while consuming large amounts of carbohydrates.

Which Diet Is Best for Me?

So, out of the three ketogenic diets, which one is best suited for you? Well, that's the difficult part. Many people find the when they are trying to find the best ketogenic diet, they often resort to trial and error. Of course, if you have a certain aim or goal with your health or physique you can choose the right diet for you depending on what that goal is.

Each of the diets that we talked about have their purposes. The standard ketogenic diet is meant to promote weight loss and even toning of the body when paired with light exercise. This can be contrasted with the purpose of the cyclic ketogenic diet where the goal is to work hard on your carb-loading days to gain muscle, while burning fat on those days that you follow the standard ketogenic diet.

Of course, the targeted ketogenic diet is a middle ground. You would choose this method if you are just beginning to gain muscle. Instead of pumping yourself full of carbs to gain muscle when you may not know how it treats your body, you can try just eating carbs before you work out. This will give you a good insider look at how you would fair if you did decide to train further someday.

So, if you are trying to gain muscle and tone your body, the cyclic ketogenic may be the best thing for you. However, if you have decided that all you want to do is lose weight and tone your body, light exercise and the standard ketogenic diet may be your best bet. This way, you would have to save yourself all the strain, planning, and counting of carbs that the cyclic diet would entail.

You should choose which type of diet is good for you based on what you want to do with your body and what you feel you need to improve on.

The Benefits of the Keto Diets

We know that the ketogenic diet promotes weight loss and muscle gain depending on how you do it. But what else does the keto diet have to offer you? Well, there are many different things that the ketogenic diet can do for your body. This includes treat diabetes, improve blood pressure, quicken metabolism, and has also been proven to improve brain function. However, there is much more!

Stress and Anti-Aging

This diet has been proven to have some effect in the aging process. This is because it has also proven to lower stress levels. This kind of emotional distress is known to "speed up cellular aging", meaning that it literally makes you look older. Stress can cause hair loss, weight gain, and the premature wrinkling of skin.

Along with this, lowering your stress levels is one way to increase your lifespan due to the decrease of insulin levels. High insulin levels mean that your body is breaking down a lot of sugars. This may be a sign that your eating habits are not as good as they should be. This could lead to obesity and could increase your chances of heart or cardiac problems and type two diabetes.

Decreases the Risk of Type 2 Diabetes

We've discussed already that the whole point of the ketogenic diet is to increase the levels of the ketones in your body. This will cause your body to burn fat instead of sugar to get energy. So how is this tied to your chances of getting type two diabetes?

Simple carbohydrates often turn to sugars when you eat them in excess. Excess sugar in the body can cause the pancreas to overwork, potentially damaging the organ. This can cause adult onset diabetes, or type two diabetes.

The ketogenic diet is just one of the easiest ways that you can reduce your chances of getting this disorder. While diabetes is a completely manageable disorder, and you can live normally with it when you manage it correctly. However, it would mean that you've damaged your body to the point where it cannot be repaired. To avoid this—especially if you have a history of diabetes in your family—it is a good idea to reduce your intake of carbohydrates and try out the ketogenic diet.

Metabolic Syndrome

Have you ever thought that maybe your metabolism is too slow? Maybe that's why you can't keep those extra ten pounds off? Well, if you do find that you have a slow metabolism, this diet may be the best for you.

It has been proven that the ketogenic diet can improve and quicken your metabolism by a staggering amount.

This is because your body is more efficient, as it burns fat for energy instead of simply sugars.

Metabolic syndrome isn't just about your body's metabolism; it is about cardiac function and your cholesterol levels. Well, the ketogenic diet can help you with all those things, along with illuminating belly fat.

The ketogenic diet is one that is built on the idea of increased fats and decreased carbs, right? Well, research shows that high blood sugar, high blood pressure, high LDL cholesterol and low HDL cholesterol can all be reduced by the reduction of carbohydrates and the addition of fats in your diet.

Acne Treatment

In recent years, research has been carried out to prove whether acne and high glycemic foods (foods high in sugar content) relate to acne breakouts. By this logic and the fact that the ketogenic diet reframes from such foods, any acne problems that you may have can be fixed or greatly improve simply by follow this diet!

Manage Hunger

So many people find that the single worst thing about being on a diet is being hungry. Unfortunately, this one of the main reasons why people do not stick with their diets and end up binging at some point.

However, the ketogenic diet proves that not all diets are difficult and temporary.

Studies have been consistently showing that a diet rich in fat and protein and low in carbohydrates can curb your hunger. This is because the food that have a higher fat content are known to have less calories in comparison to foods that have a lot of carbohydrates. In other words, you will be able to eat more for less, allowing you to ensure that you can be full all day long!

Along with this, researchers have found that to compare low-carb and low-fat diets, they must "actively restrict calories in the low-fat groups."

Maintaining of Body Weight

You may find that once you lose weight, you may end up gaining is back again. This causes you to try again. You lose more weight and you gain more back. That is what many people call yo-yo dieting and it can be very hazardous to your health.

To avoid this from happening, it is advised that you make a diet a lifestyle change instead of just a temporary thing. The research shows that the ketogenic diet is one of the best and easiest to maintain. This means that dedicating some time and effort into the lifestyle change, you can keep your weight where you want it to be.

Chapter Two: Getting Started

So, we know what the keto diet is, we know what it does to our body and we know how useful it is, but how do we go about actually starting the diet? Well, there are a few things that you are advised to do before you begin to ensure that you succeed. It is also a good idea to take body measurements and get a proper check up with the doctor to get a feel of where your body is right now in terms of health. This can help you in the long run when you may want to go back and look at how far you have come.

Before You Begin the Diet

What do you do before you begin any diet? You take some before and after pictures and you check out your measurements, but this may not be as easy for some people. Many people find it difficult to find the correct places to measure, and a lot of people are too ashamed to take a before photo. Let's deal with those problems first, head on.

Taking Your Measurements

Before being a diet, you could always take and write down your measurements and weight so that you can look back on it during your journey to see just how far you have come. Some people find it difficult, however, to take their measurements in the right places and many other people do not know all the places they should be taking their measurements.

Let's begin with the different places you should measure.

Most of the time, the most important places that you want to measure are your hips, waist, and bust. When measuring your hips, you should be aiming to find the widest part of your hip bone. That would usually be about two inches below your belly button. Your waist is the smallest, most narrow part of your torso. It is usually found just above your belly button. Measuring your bust usually entails lining your tape measure up with your nipples. For men, you can measure just under your nipples to get a chest measurement instead. There usually isn't much of a difference; it is completely up to you.

You will also find that measuring the legs and arms are useful, as well. There are two different places that you can measure on your legs. It's up to you whether you measure both and which one you want to measure. Most often, people measure their thighs and calves; their thighs being the fullest part of your leg when you are standing and your calves being the fullest part of your lower leg. For your arms, people usually just measure their upper arm which is the fullest part of your arm above the elbow.

Taking Your Before Photo

Taking a before picture may be difficult sometimes for two main reasons. When you have self-esteem issues due to your weight or even the shape of your body, you may not find it very comfortable taking a picture of your body in just your underwear. Secondly, when you haven't taken pictures like these before, you may not really know what to do with your body or how to pose.

First, for those who may not want to have photos of you in your underwear on your phone or computer and some people may just not want to see those pictures, there are a few things that you can do to help yourself with these problems. When you take your picture, you could simply not even bother with taking it in your underwear. A good idea is to take your photos in a pair of short and a strap shirt. This may be more comfortable for those who do not want to take the half nude photos. Even though the pictures are only for you, it just might make you feel exposed. If you really want to take the photos in your underwear but you are afraid of someone finding them on your phone, you can find many apps on both Android and Apple app stores that act as a picture and document "vault." It will keep your photos from being found.

Another thing to worry about when you take your pictures is how you pose your body. This is very simple! The best pose you could try is putting your feet together with your hands down at your sides. You should also take a sideways picture where you can see your buttocks and sides. Here, you would have your arms at or sides or up in the air and your feet together.

You may find it easier to get someone else to take the picture but if not, standing in front of a full-length mirror should suffice.

Finding Your Ideal Body Weight and BMI

Another thing that you may find useful is to know your ideal weight for your height and age. Unfortunately, there is no way that we can calculate this number using simple math, but there are many websites on the internet that can calculate a good number for you. For example, a woman that is 25 years old and is 5 feet 6 inches may be most healthy in the 115 lbs to 155 lbs range. It is important to know, however, that these numbers are just a guide. It is not recommended to starve yourself or lose weight by any unhealthy means to achieve these goals.
You may also want to calculate your BMI or body mass index. Your body mass index is a measurement of whether you are at a healthy weight. Calculating your BMI is quick and easy. You can do this one manually, but you can find websites on the internet that can do all the work for you.

Begin by changing your weight into kilograms. You can then go ahead and change your height into meters. Divide your weight in kilograms by your height in meters, and then divide what you get for that by your height in meters again. This should give you your BMI. You can check on a BMI chart to see if you are at a healthy weight for your height.

Here is an example of a person that is 150 pounds at a height of 5 foot 6:

150 lbs = 68 kg

5 feet 6 inches = 1.67 m

68 kg divided by 1.67m is equal to 40.7

40.7 divided by 1.67 is equal to 24.4.

This person's BMI is 24.4.

Determine Your Recommended Daily Calorie Intake

If you find out your recommended daily calorie intake—found from your body weight, height, and age—you can find out exactly how many calories you should be eating in a day to A) lose weight B) maintain your weight or C) gain weight. There are many online calculators, just like the ideal weight and BMI calculators that you can find.

Talk to your Doctor

It may be a good idea to talk to your doctor before you begin any sort of lifestyle change. People say this but have you really considered why going to the doctor is so important?

Well, consulting your doctor before beginning a new diet or trying to lose weight may be a good idea because you will get the chance to have a talk with a professional and get the most realistic goal for your body type. Your doctor may even help you by giving you advice or directing you to a dietician or nutritionist that can help you plan your meals and advise you on what you can do to optimize your weight loss.

Of course, checking for any health problems may be a good idea as well. You do not want to make any drastic changes to your body and end up damaging it.

Prepare Your Pantry

Before we talk about what foods you are looking to buy when you start your ketogenic diet, you should sort your pantry out. It is a good idea to take all the foods you want to avoid and put it to one side. If you have a family this is especially important, but if you live alone, you can take the food out of your home all together, if you wish. You don't have to throw it away; donating it or giving it to a family member or friend will be much better than wasting the food.

If you have a family—or if you live with a roommate— you may find it difficult to stay out of the junk food or the foods rich in carbohydrates. When times like these come up, you must remember that you are strong. You need to remember that you are doing this to be a better, healthier you. If it helps, you can ask your roommate to take their junk food into their room or hide it away. You can also ask your family or roommate to watch after you and help you make sure that you don't make any decisions that you may regret.

The Pace of your Diet

Before you begin, you should decide how fast you want your diet to progress. You can choose from one of two speeds or paces, those being the obvious fast and slow.

Fast pace entails for the abrupt drop of carbohydrates, cold turkey. This may be the harder option, but it is the "rip-off-the-band-aid" method where you just get it over with. You wake up one morning and swear to have a few eggs and some yogurt for breakfast instead of toast. It is on that day that you swear off carbs (assuming you are following the standard ketogenic diet) for as long as you possibly can. No breaks, no "treats."

People find the fast pace method a little harder because they drop everything and tend to miss it more. However, there is a way around it. You can take the slower paced method. This method means that you would gradually exclude carbohydrates from your diet. It is a lot easier because you don't have to give up the foods you love right away—you wean yourself off them as you please. There are still some risks with this method, though. You may not wean yourself off the foods fast enough or you may end up cheating. In other words, this method may seem a little slack to most people.

While the choice is completely up to you, as it is based off your preferences, your willpower, and your needs, it is very strongly recommended that you do the fast pace method first.

What should you expect?

With most diets, you will begin to see a difference in your body right away. However, with the ketogenic diet you may see a few changes that you may not expect. Because this diet has a lot to do with the chemical processes and mechanisms in your body, there will be some significant but small changes that will be noticed. Some of these include muscle cramps, the feeling of tiredness, bad breath, frequent urination, and what we call "keto flu."

Though most of those are self explanatory, or you've experienced them in the past, the keto flu is most likely new to you.

Keto flu is a bundle of symptoms that you experience when you change to a low carb diet. The symptoms often include tiredness, dizziness, cravings for bread, pasta and sugary substances and difficulty staying focused. Keto flu is known for occurring in people who have cut a lot of carbs out of their diet and is known as both keto flu and carb flu.

You don't have to worry, keto flu is not that bad, and it doesn't affect everybody that gives up carbs. It usually only last about a week or two, however, if you are "lucky enough" you may experience it for longer; it is different in everyone.

Fixing or getting rid of keto flu may be as easy as drinking more water, eating more fat and complex carbs (vegetables and fruit), eating more calories, eating more salt or exercising more. However, it may be a little more difficult than that for you. The best way to get rid of it is to keep doing what you're doing and power through. Just remember that you want this.

Chapter Three: What to Eat, What to Eat...

As with most diets, there is a semi-strict shopping list that you are advised to follow to get success with this diet. We already know that carbs are supposed to be cut out, but what exactly are we to cut out? Let's have a look!

A Little Bit About Carbs

Carbohydrates are "very controversial" these days (authoritynutrition.com). Some people say that we should eat plenty of carbs, while others say that they are bad for you and can cause type two diabetes and obesity. And the thing is: both are correct. "But how is that?" you ask. Well, let's have a look at the three-different kind of carbs that there are.

Some carbohydrates are sugars in disguise. These are "short-chained" carbohydrates that are usually found in foods. You may know these guys as fructose, glucose, and sucrose. Most of these sugars are the ones that we were told by the nutritionist to avoid, right? And your nutritionist has never been more right. These are refined sugars, those that are the worst for you, and bad for building fat around the belly.

Other carbohydrates hide in our bread, bagels, cereal and the ever so delicious pasta. Who doesn't love a good pasta? Well, unfortunately, pasta isn't your friend; in fact, pasta may be the reason why you have that little bit of extra pudge hanging out on your abdomen. It is known that these sorts of carbs are often converted right to sugar when they begin to digest. These are the carbs that you really want to steer clear from, as they are the ones that block the ketones from burning fat for energy.

Finally, we have fiber. Yes, fiber is a carbohydrate. However, it is a much better carbohydrate. It should be known that humans don't even digest fiber; it either goes right through you, or the "friendly bacteria" in the digestive system eat it up and use it as fuel.

So, you can see that there are carbs that are easy to break down—they are much more simple—and there are carbohydrates that are broken down with much more difficulty—or not at all. That brings us to whole and refined carbs.

Also, known as simple and complex carbohydrates, "whole" and "refined" are just words that we can further use to describe carbohydrates based on their condition *before* they go into the body.

"Whole carbs are unprocessed" and there is fiber found naturally in the food while refined carbs are known to be processed and the natural has been "stripped out". Whole carbohydrates are usually in foods that are described as healthy. This includes whole fruits (apples, tomatoes, peaches, watermelon, etc), vegetables, and whole grains. These foods are the ones that you want to restrict but still eat in moderation (about 50-60 grams a day at the most).

What Else?

It is very important that the foods you eat are not processed in anyway. Processed foods often led to processed carbohydrates, therefore you will want to stay away from them to be as successful as possible.

Enough about the foods that you should avoid; what can you eat?

Depending on your regular eating habits, meats that are not processed, healthy fats, vegetables, fruits (whole fruit), full fat yogurt and cheese, drink that are not sugary and nuts and seeds. As you can see, there is no shortage of foods that you can eat and you will not go hungry!

Meats

Since you want to eat lots of healthy fats and protein, you should make sure that you are eating organic, non-processed meats daily. Most health guides say that you should be eating at least one portion (about 3 ounces) of meat daily.

However, you'll want to stay away from processed meats. This can include the following:

- Sausages and hot dogs
- Chicken nuggets and patties
- Bologna
- Pepperoni and salami
- Spam
- Canned meats (excluding tuna and salmon)
- Bacon

There are many more but these are the most common processed meats that you may run into. When you are looking for healthy meats to buy, make sure that you aim for meats that are freshly cut at your grocery store. Meats like ribs, steaks, pork chops and boneless and skinless chicken breast are all wonderful for the ketogenic diet.

It is recommended that you eat plenty of chicken and turkey. Both poultries are great for you and there are many things that you can substitute as chicken or turkey. For example, you'll notice that ground beef is quite greasy and may be bad for you if you eat it in excess—even though it is so yummy. However, you can trade it in for extra lean ground turkey. This still may not be healthy, but it is much better than the greasy mess that you get from ground beef.

Healthy Fats

So, we've been talking about fats and how the keto diet requires a lot of them. "But won't fat make me fat?" Absolutely not! When we talk about eating fats, we mean that you should eat plenty of healthy or "good" fats. So why exactly are those good fats?

Well good fats are recommended in your daily diet and the normal adult should know that 20% to 35% of your daily calories should come from fat. However, the problem isn't that people aren't eating enough fat, it's that they are not eating the right ones. Roughly 35% to 40% of our daily calorie intake is fat but not the right ones. This can cause our waistlines to expand and can increase your overall risk of type two diabetes and heart problems.

So, which fats are the best ones to eat? You can find "good for you fats" in many of the meats that you eat— assuming that they are grass fed and are fresh. Good fats are also found in avocado, coconut, almonds, dark chocolate, flax and chia seeds, tuna and salmon, and eggs.

Vegetables

There aren't many rules when it comes to vegetables and the ketogenic diet, however, you'll want to stick with above ground vegetables and leafy greens. It really doesn't matter if the vegetables are fresh or frozen, but when it comes to what tastes better, we always recommend fresh.

Some of the vegetables you should be aiming for include the following:

- Lettuce
- Spinach
- Cabbage
- Asparagus
- Tomato
- Broccoli
- Green, red and yellow peppers
- Beans
- Kale
- Eggplants

This is just a short list of many, many vegetable that you can add to your diet to ensure that you get enough of the nutrients that your body needs to function correctly, lose weight and get healthy. However, you are advised to stay away from legumes.

Fruit

It is well known that fruit contains plenty of natural sugars. It is because of this that you should avoid eating a lot of fruit. However, there are lots of fruit that you can still eat to satisfy your sweet tooth without blowing your diet.

We all know just how sour lemons are, so it wouldn't surprise you that they do not contain a whole lot of sugar. That's right you can still drink your lemon water or enjoy happy hour with a lemon wedge. Along with lemons, you can still indulge in some sweet and delicious strawberries. Strawberries are surprisingly low in sugar and are actually packed full of vitamin C.

In fact, many berries are low in sugar. This includes raspberries and blackberries. That means that you can still enjoy your morning smoothie and you won't be going off track. Remember, though, they may be low in sugar but many fruit mentioned here still have a nice amount. Just be careful not to eat too much.

Here is a list of fruits that you can indulge in every now and then:

- Lemons
- Limes
- Raspberries
- Strawberries
- Blackberries
- Kiwis
- Grapefruit
- Avocado
- Watermelon
- Oranges
- Peaches

Enjoy! But remember to keep it slow when it comes to fruit. You don't want to avoid carbohydrates just to eat more sugar.

Dairy

When it comes to dairy, you want to avoid from drinking too much milk, but you'll also want to embrace full fat Greek yogurt. Greek yogurt is known to have plenty of those good fats along with plenty or protein, making it good for your bones, muscles, cartilage, skin, hair and blood. Protein help you provide energy, while you will burn the fat for more energy during ketosis.

You can sneak some "fake dairy" into your everyday life as well. Coconut and almond milk is really good for you and give you the fats that you're looking for with the ketogenic diet. You can add either one of these beverages to smoothies, substitute them in recipes and use them in your cereal in the morning if you really wanted to illuminate cow's milk.

Chapter Four: Recipes

Breakfast

Breakfast is one of the best and most important meals of the day, so it is very important that you make sure you are getting all the nutrients that you need so that you can power through your day like a champion. Even when you are on a diet, you should make sure that your breakfast is large and will last you right up until lunch, no matter what you'll have to face in those few hours before you get to refuel.

Cheese Omelet

This is a simple, yet delicious cheese omelet that you can master quickly and still get enough fuel to keep you going all morning! Who doesn't love a good, old classic breakfast? It should be noted that this recipe is enough for two people, so if you are dining alone, you can just half the few ingredients.

Ingredients
- 1 teaspoon of butter
- 6 eggs
- 7 ounces of shredded cheddar cheese (or whichever you prefer)
- Salt and pepper to taste

Directions

1. Beat the eggs in a bowl—make sure they are slightly frothy—and throw in half of the shredded cheese in the bowl with them. You may also add salt and pepper as you like.
2. Warm a pan on medium heat and melt your butter. At this point in time, once the butter has melted completely, you can pour in your egg and cheese mixture.
3. Turn down the heat on your pan and let the eggs sit for a moment. Wait until they are almost completely cooked through.
4. Add the rest of the cheese on top of the egg and let it melt. Allow the egg to cook right through, at this time as well.
5. Fold your omelet over and serve hot.

It's good to know that you can spice up your omelet by adding in whatever you'd like. Some people like green, red, or yellow peppers in their omelets, others like mushrooms and herbs. You can do whatever you like with this dish. That is why it is a favorite among so many people.

Low-Carb Frittata with Spinach

This delicious and beautiful looking dish is a wonderful one to serve when you have friends or family over for a visit and you don't know what to get for breakfast. This recipe—like the other is made for more people, so you may have left overs. You can also double, half, or quarter the dish to your liking. This recipe serves four people.

Ingredients
- 8 eggs
- 1 cup of heavy whipping cream
- 1/2 lb. of fresh spinach
- 1/3 lb. of diced bacon or chorizo
- 1/3 lb. shredded cheese (whatever kind you prefer)
- 2 tablespoons of butter (for frying)
- Salt and pepper to taste

Directions
1. Start by preheating your oven to 350°F.
2. Fry your bacon in the butter on medium heat until it is crispy. Once it's finished, add your spinach to the bacon in the pan and let it cook.
3. Beat the eggs and cream together in a bowl. Here you can add salt and pepper as you please. Add this mixture to a greased baking dish.
4. Sprinkle the spinach and bacon mixture and the cheese on top of the egg and place it in the oven (the middle will give you the best results).
5. Bake for about 25 to 30 minutes and serve when hot.

Eggs Butter with Smoked Salmon and Avocado

This is called the "breakfast for champions." It will give you enough energy to face the morning with the power pose of a life time. This breakfast is not difficult at all, either! There is one thing, though: you choose to buy smoked salmon from the store, or you can choose to do this at home separately from this recipe. It is completely up to you; either way, it is going to be delicious.

Ingredients
- 4 eggs
- 1/2 teaspoon ground black pepper
- 5 ounces of butter (at room temperature)
- 2 avocados
- 2 tablespoons of olive oil
- 1 tablespoon of fresh parsley
- 4 ounces of smoked salmon

Directions
1. Place your eggs in a pot (be careful not to break them) and cover them with cold water. Lay the pot on a burner and allow to come to a boil.
2. Once the water is boiling, lower the heat and let it simmer for seven to eight minutes. After that, you can remove the eggs from the warm water and put them in ice cold water to cool (so that you can peel them).
3. After letting them cool, you can peel the eggs and chop them into small pieces. Milk the butter and

eggs together and season with the pepper and salt to taste. Here is where you can add in some other things as you please.

4. Serve the egg butter with a side of diced avocado tossed in olive oil, finely chopped parsley, and a few slices of warmed (or cold) smoked salmon.

Egg Muffins

Ingredients
- 1 or 2 scallions, finely chopped
- 3 1/2 ounces of shredded cheese
- 1 tablespoons of red or green pesto (depending on what you like)—this is optional
- Salt and pepper to taste

Directions
1. Preheat your oven to 350°F.
2. Take your scallions and whisk the eggs together with seasoning and the pesto. Add the cheese and mix them together.
3. Place your "batter" in muffin forms in a tray and bake for 15 to 20 minutes.

Chicken and Zucchini Breakfast Quiche

This meal is great in terms of prep work. The crust is something that you can pre-make and freeze, you can make it fresh or you can buy a pre-made pie crust from your local grocery store. Other than that, it's like you're making a giant omelet.

Ingredients
- Crust:
    - 2 cups of almond flour
    - 2 tablespoons of coconut oil
    - A pinch of sea salt
    - 1 large egg
- Filling:
    - 6 large eggs
    - 1/2 cup of heavy cream
    - 1 or 2 medium zucchinis (grated)
    - 1 tablespoon fennel seed
    - 1 teaspoon dried oregano
    - 1 teaspoon salt
    - 1/2 teaspoon black pepper
    - 1 lb. ground chicken

Directions
1. Preheat your oven to 350°F.
2. For the crust, you just have to mix (in a food processor) the almond flour and salt. Then you can add in the coconut oil and egg with it. The mixture should form a ball.

3. From there, you can take the mixture out and flatten it out into a lightly greased 9-inch pie dish and set aside. You do not have to pre-bake this crust.
4. Cook the ground chicken first in a large skillet.
5. In a large bowl, beat the eggs until smooth. Add the cream and spices and stir really well. Mix in the grated zucchini and cooled chicken. Make sure everything is coated in egg and pour into the pie crust.
6. Bake for 30-40 minutes or until the center is firm and the crust is golden.

Lunch

Research has shown that, even though breakfast should be your biggest meal of the day, lunch should be a close second. This is because around noon is where your day usually picks up. So, even though breakfast is the most important meal of the day, a good, hearty lunch is a good idea, especially if you work or if you're a student.

Healthy Tuna Stuffed Avocado

Stuffed avocado is one of the quickest lunches that you can come up with. It's something that you can mix up and put together at work the next day. This is also one of the healthiest things that you could put in your body. Both tuna and avocado are known to be notoriously healthy for you, providing you with healthy fats and lots of protein.

Ingredients
- 1 avocado, halved and pitted
- 1 can of tuna, drained
- 1/4 cups of diced red bell pepper
- 1 tablespoon of minced jalapeño
- 1/4 cup of cilantro leaves, roughly chopped
- 1 tablespoon of lime juice
- Salt and pepper to taste

Directions

1. Scoop out some of the avocado after pitting it to make more room. Put the scooped-out avocado in a mixing bowl.
2. Add the tuna, chopped bell pepper, jalapeño, and cilantro to the mixing bowl and pour the lime juice over it. Mush and mix everything together, making sure it is all combined.
3. Put the mixture into the scooped-out places in the avocado halves. Season it with salt.

If you are looking to bring this lunch to school or work, it is best to do steps one and two home and then add the tuna mixture to your avocado when you are ready to eat it.

Keto BLT Salad

Ingredients
- Dressing
    - 1/4 cup of mayonnaise
    - 2 teaspoons of lemon juice
    - 2 teaspoons of apple cider vinegar (or water)
    - 4 to 10 drops of pure liquid stevia (to taste)
- Salad
    - 2 cups of chopped romaine lettuce
    - 1/4 lb. of good quality bacon (you can use turkey bacon)
    - 1/2 a medium tomato, chopped

Directions
1. Whisk together all the ingredients for the dressing in a small or medium mixing bowl.
2. In a separate, larger bowl mix together your salad ingredients, adding in the dressing and mixing together.

Simple, huh? It's a quick recipe that you can whip up before you go to bed. Just store your dressing in a separate container and mix right before eating. This is the perfect salty treat to reward yourself for a good week or a good month. Enjoy!

Low Carb Salmon Fish Cakes

Ingredients
- 2 cans of pink salmon
- 2 teaspoons chopped chives
- 1/4 cup of chopped dill
- 1/4 cup of grated parmesan cheese
- 4 ounces of pork rinds, crushed
- 2 large eggs
- 1 teaspoon of lemon zest
- Salt and pepper to taste
- 1/2 cup of almond flour
- 2 tablespoons of olive oil

Directions
1. Open and drain both cans of salmon into a large mixing bowl.
   Add the chives, dill, cheese, crushed pork rinds, eggs, lemon zest and the salt and pepper to the salmon.
2. Next, you can form the salmon into three ounce balls. This usually ends up forming ten balls.
3. Pour some of the almond flour onto a plate or in a bowl, flatten each ball and dip it in the almond flour. Make sure to tap all the excess flour off the salmon.
4. Preheat a skillet with two tablespoons of olive oil. The frying pan should be at a medium to high heat. Cook the salmon on each side for a few minutes each.
5. Serve with tartar sauce and vegetables.

Cauliflower Bread

Ingredients
- 1 medium head of cauliflower
- Parchment paper
- Nonstick cooking spray
- Cheese cloth
- 1 large egg
- 1/2 cup of shredded mozzarella cheese

Directions
1. Preheat oven to 400 degrees.
2. Line a large baking sheet with parchment paper and lightly coat it with non-stick spray.
3. Cut the cauliflower in half and place one of the halves in a food processor and pulse until it is the size of rice grains. Repeat with other half.
4. Transfer to a microwave safe bowl and place in microwave on high for six to eight minutes or until the cauliflower is fully cooked.
5. Place the cooked cauliflower on cheese cloth in small batches and squeeze dry, make sure you squeeze as much water out as you can.
6. Transfer, again, to a bowl and mix in the egg, cheese, salt, and pepper.
7. Place the cauliflower on the parchment paper in squares and bake for 15 to 17 minutes.
8. Make sure to let them cool for about 10 minutes before removing them from the baking sheet (carefully).

Dinner

Ah, dinner. A time when you can sit down with your family and friends and talk about your day. But every night you wonder what you're going to cook. Why is it so difficult to get a good, healthy meal—that everyone can enjoy—on the table every night? Well, you don't have to struggle anymore! We have some wonderfully easy—and kid friendly—meals that you and your family can enjoy.

Chicken Broccoli Casserole

Have you ever just wanted to get something ready, shove it in the oven and forget about it for a while? Well, this is the meal for you! Cooking it is easy as pie and you can get it done in no time. The best part of this casserole is the fact that you can hide the broccoli with the cheese. Kid friendly? I think so.

Ingredients
- 2 tablespoons of coconut oil
- 4 cups of fresh broccoli
- 1 medium white onion, diced
- Salt and pepper to taste
- 8 ounces of mushrooms, sliced
- 3 cups of cooked chicken, shredded
- 1 cup of chicken broth
- 1 cup of full fat coconut milk
- 2 eggs
- 2 cups of shredded cheese (optional)

- 1/2 teaspoon of nutmeg (optional)

Directions
1. Preheat your oven to 350°F.
2. Grease a casserole dish with some of the coconut oil and set aside.
3. Steam the broccoli until it is just starting to cook and set aside while you melt the rest of the coconut oil and brown the onions in a frying pan. You can now season it with salt and pepper however you like.
4. Add the mushrooms to the sauce pan and let cook. Add the shredded chicken, broccoli, mushrooms, and onions to the casserole dish. Make sure everything is evenly distributed within the pan.
5. Mix the broth, cheese, eggs, coconut milk, nutmeg and a generous pinch of salt and pepper in a separate bowl. Poor this mixture into the casserole dish evenly.
6. Put the dish into the oven for about 35 to 40 minutes.

As you can see, this is a pretty family friendly meal and is easy to prepare. There isn't really any peeling or preparing of the vegetables and the ingredients are not difficult to get. This meal is so great because you can basically throw the ingredients in and go about your business.

Barbecue Bacon Cheddar Meatloaf

Ingredients
- Meatloaf
  - 2 lbs. of ground beef (you can use ground turkey)
  - 1 cup of shredded cheddar
  - 1 tablespoon of dried minced onion
  - 1 teaspoon of dried minced garlic
  - 1 teaspoon of garlic powder
  - 1 teaspoon of ground mustard
  - 1 teaspoon of chili power
  - 1 teaspoon of salt
  - 2 ounces of sugar free barbecue sauce
  - 1 egg
- Toppings
  - 2 ounces of sugar free barbecue sauce
  - 1/2 cup of shredded cheddar cheese
  - 1/2 cup of cooked chopped bacon (about 5 slices)

Directions
1. Preheat your oven to 400°F.
2. Combine all the ingredients for the meatloaf into one large mixing bowl and press into a 9 by 13 casserole dish.
3. Brush the 2 ounces of barbecue sauce you saved on top of the meat and sprinkle on the cheese and then the bacon.

Meatloaf is not only a good band, but it is also a very versatile meal. You can put pretty much whatever you like in meatloaf. For example, you may find that you like lots of peppers in your meatloaf or you may be like some people add ketchup or tomato sauce.

Meatloaf is also a great meal in the way that you can pair it with anything. For instance, you can pair is with mashed potatoes, rice, mixed vegetables or even some French fries for the kids.

Turkey Taco Lettuce Wraps

If you absolutely love tacos, like so many of us, but hate the stomach ache you get after you "accidentally" eat four or five, then you will absolutely love this recipe. This alteration to the traditional tortilla or hard shell tacos will let you eat the same number of tacos while decreasing the amount of carbs *and* calories.

Ingredients
- 1 lb. 95% lean ground turkey
- 1 tablespoon of olive oil
- 3/4 cup onion, finely chopped
- Salt and pepper to taste
- 1 tablespoon chili powder
- 1 teaspoon of ground cumin
- 1/2 teaspoon of paprika
- 1/2 cup of tomato sauce
- 2 cloves of garlic
- 1/2 cup low-sodium chicken broth
- Iceberg or romaine lettuce leaves
- Shredded cheese (whichever kind you like)
- Diced tomatoes
- Diced red onion
- Chopped cilantro
- Light sour cream

Directions
1. Heat the olive oil in a non-stick skillet over medium heat.

2. Add the onion and cook until transparent. Add the turkey, garlic, salt, and pepper and cook. Make sure to break up the ground turkey into smaller pieces, while waiting for the turkey to cook completely through (about five minutes).
3. Once it is cooked through, add the tomato sauce, chili powder, paprika, cumin, and chicken broth. Lower the heat to simmer, and cook this for about five minutes until the sauce is reduced.
4. Serve the mixture in the lettuce leaves using the desired toppings.

Buttery Lemon Chicken

Ingredients
- 4 chicken breasts, skinless and boneless
- 1/3 cup chicken broth
- 1 teaspoon Italian seasoning
- 3 tablespoons of butter
- 1 tablespoons of honey
- 2 tablespoons of minced garlic
- 4 tablespoons of fresh lemon juice
- Salt and pepper to taste
- Fresh rosemary and lemon slices for garnish (optional)

Directions
1. Preheat your oven to 400 degrees and grease a large casserole dish.
2. Melt the butter in a large pan on medium heat and add the chicken. Cook for two to three minutes on each side or until they are browned. Put chicken into the casserole dish.
3. Whisk together the chicken broth, Italian seasoning, honey, lemon juice, garlic, and salt and pepper in a small bowl.
4. Pour the mixture over the chicken and bake for 20 to 30 minutes or until the chicken is completely cooked through. Make sure that you spoon the sauce over the chicken every five to ten minutes.
5. Garnish with fresh rosemary and lemon slices if desired and serve hot.

Turkey Soup

Ingredients
- 1 turkey leg or left overs from a 10 to 12-pound turkey
- 2 quarts of water
- 1 medium onion, cut in wedges
- 1/2 teaspoon of salt
- 2 bay leaves
- 1 cup of chopped carrots
- 1 cup of uncooked long grain rice
- 1/3 cup of chopped celery
- 1/4 cup of chopped onion
- 1 can (10 3/4 ounces) of cream of chicken soup

Directions
1. Place all your turkey into a large pot and add the onion, bay leaves, salt and water and let it boil. Let the turkey cook for about 2 hours.
2. Remove all or at least most of the bones, large onions and bay leaves. Add the rice, carrots, celery, and chopped onions. Cover and let the vegetables and rice get tender.
3. Add the cream soup and let warm up.

Chapter Five: 30 Day Meal Plan

Now that we know what to do before we start the keto diet, and we know what kind of foods we should be eating we can begin the diet. Let's look at a 30-day meal plan that you can follow to be as successful as you possibly can.

Learning from a sample meal plan will help you get use to and learn how to cook for yourself and your family without the help of a diet plan. So let's get started.

Even though there are two different paces that you can set your diet at, we recommend the fast pace method, so that is how we are going to do it here. There are small modifications that you can make to set this meal plan to your liking.

Week One

Sunday

Breakfast: three egg omelet with peppers, mushrooms, and onions with 1 cup of raspberries and strawberries (mixed) with full-fat Greek yogurt.
Lunch: salad with tomatoes, cheese, bacon bits (real) and organic ham dressed with an olive oil, vinegar, and lemon dressing.
Snack: one apple and a small chunk of cheddar cheese. (Tip: take a bite of the apple and then cheese. Chew together—it tastes amazing).

Dinner: here, you can try your chicken broccoli casserole.

Monday

Breakfast: 2 egg muffins with a tall glass of milk (coconut, almond, or cow's).
Lunch: tuna salad, made with mayonnaise, avocado, onions, and celery paired with whole grain crackers.
Snack: one cup of full-fat Greek yogurt with raspberries.
Dinner: turkey taco lettuce wraps.

Tuesday

Breakfast: full-fat yogurt with granola and fruit (whichever that are ketogenic diet friendly).
Lunch: stuffed avocados.
Snack: a handful of almond (or any nut that you prefer).
Dinner: turkey soup.

Wednesday

Breakfast: three scrambled eggs with half an avocado.
Lunch: classic Caesar salad with a side of sliced avocado (the leftover half from breakfast).
Snack: a cup of mixed raspberries and strawberries.
Dinner: barbecue bacon meatloaf.

Thursday

Breakfast: low carb frittata with spinach.
Lunch: chicken caesar wrap with croutons!
Snack: one orange and full fat Greek yogurt.
Dinner: low carb salmon fish cakes.

Friday

Breakfast: breakfast wrap (two eggs, organic ham, and cheese).
Lunch: one cup of full-fat Greek yogurt mixed with almonds (or any nut that you prefer), granola, and any ketogenic friendly fruit that you want.
Snack: small chunk of cheese with whole wheat crackers.
Dinner: steak and keto BLT salad.

Saturday

Breakfast: eggs butter, smoked salmon, and avocado.
Lunch: chef salad.
Snack: dark chocolate and strawberries.
Dinner: stuffed chicken breast with steamed vegetables.

Week Two

This week, we want to try to wean off our snacks. Just eating breakfast, lunch and dinner will have a fasting effect. You may feel hungry at first, but your body will slowly get used to it.

Sunday

Breakfast: two scrambled eggs and a slice of whole wheat toast with any kind of nut butter that you prefer.
Lunch: chicken Caesar wrap with cheese and a glass of milk (which ever kind you prefer).
Snack: one orange and a cup of yogurt.
Dinner: steak with sweet potatoes, asparagus and steamed broccoli

Monday

Breakfast: breakfast smoothie! 1 cup of strawberries, 1 cup of raspberries, 1/2 a cup of full-fat Greek yogurt and 1 cup of milk (whichever kind you prefer).
Lunch: salad with tomatoes, lettuce, spinach, bacon bits (real), red onion, red, yellow and/or green peppers and your choice of dressing.
Snack: one apple
Dinner: barbecue chicken breast with chicken (or turkey) wieners, fried mushrooms and onions, and baked potato.

Tuesday

Breakfast: avocado-eggs bake (pit avocado, crack eggs into the holes and bake at 350°F until egg is cooked).
Lunch: no bread grilled cheese sandwich.
Dinner: barbecue salmon and steamed vegetables.

Wednesday

Breakfast: breakfast egg muffins.
Lunch: tuna salad with whole wheat crackers.
Dinner: chef salad with tomatoes, chicken, red onions, and peppers (any kind you like).

Thursday

Breakfast: two boiled eggs with one cup of full-fat yogurt and raspberries.
Lunch: no bread smoked salmon sandwich with lettuce, spinach, red onion and mayonnaise (sounds weird, but, trust me, it's so good).
Dinner: barbecued steak with asparagus (seasoned with butter and garlic) and corn.

Friday

Breakfast: chicken wieners, scrambled eggs, and one chicken breast (tip: it's really good if you cut up the chicken wieners and chicken breast and mix it in with your eggs).
Lunch: stuffed avocado
Dinner: chicken breast (cooked whichever way you like) and BLT salad.

Saturday

Breakfast: two boiled eggs and half an avocado.
Lunch: salmon fishcakes.
Dinner: chicken broccoli casserole.

Week Three

Now that we have eliminated all of the snacks between meals, this week we'll want to aim for more fats and high protein content. This is going to be a great week!

Sunday

Breakfast: full-fat yogurt with crushed flax seeds, two eggs (cooked however you like), with a hand full of your favorite nuts.
Lunch: summer melon fruit salad (honeydew, cantaloupe, and watermelon with grapes, and strawberries).
Dinner: chicken breast cooked however you like with steamed broccoli and pan fried asparagus (in garlic and butter).

Monday

Breakfast: two eggs, half an avocado, and smoked salmon.
Lunch: chicken and cheese wrap with lettuce, spinach, red onion, and peppers (any that you like).
Dinner: barbecue bacon meatloaf with steamed vegetable and mashed (sweet or white/red) potatoes.

Tuesday

Breakfast: one egg, the other half of the avocado from yesterday and pan fried chicken breast seasoned any way that you like it.

Lunch: tuna salad with mayonnaise, onions, peppers (of any kind), and tomatoes served with any kind of whole wheat crackers.

Dinner: philly cheese steak sandwich with cauliflower bread.

Wednesday

Breakfast: two boiled eggs.

Lunch: no bread grilled cheese sandwich.

Dinner: chicken fajitas with red, green, yellow, and jalapeño peppers seasoned with cumin, chili powder, salt, and pepper. Use any toppings that you like.

Thursday

Breakfast: one cup of full-fat yogurt with half a cup of strawberries, with 1/4 cup of granola.

Lunch: large chef salad with cheese, tomatoes, one boiled egg, organic ham, and real bacon bits with the dressing that you

Dinner: lemon chicken.

Friday

Breakfast: one breakfast muffin with a strawberry kiwi smoothie (strawberries, kiwi, full-fat yogurt, half a banana, and some milk to help it blend smooth).

Lunch: Caesar salad wrap with cheese and croutons!

Dinner: chicken and broccoli casserole

Saturday

Breakfast: eggs butter with smoked salmon and avocado.
Lunch: garden salad with whichever salad dressing you prefer.
Dinner: Boiled cod fish with mashed potatoes and butter.

Week Four

Sunday

Breakfast: cheese omelet with one cup of full-fat yogurt.
Lunch: mixed berry smoothie (strawberries, raspberries, full fat yogurt, milk for smooth mixing, and half a banana).
Dinner: cauliflower crust pizza (use the same recipe as cauliflower bread and cover with desired toppings).

Monday

Breakfast: two scrambled eggs with cauliflower bread.
Lunch: classic Caesar salad.
Dinner: barbecue bacon meatloaf.

Tuesday

Breakfast: Spinach frittata with organic ham.
Lunch: grilled cheese sandwich (with cauliflower bread).
Dinner: chicken fajitas (same as the other week).

Wednesday

Breakfast: egg muffins.
Lunch: chicken salad with mayonnaise, celery, tomatoes, cheese, red onion, and green onion.
Dinner: home-made honey glazed ham.

Thursday

Breakfast: watermelon, cantaloupe, honeydew, strawberry, and kiwi fruit salad with full-fat yogurt.
Lunch: BLT salad.
Dinner: turkey soup.

Friday

Breakfast: two boiled eggs with half an avocado
Lunch: stuffed avocado (the leftover half from breakfast) and one cup of full fat yogurt.
Dinner: lemon chicken.

Saturday

Breakfast: two slices of cauliflower bead and one boiled egg with a big glass of milk.
Lunch: chicken Caesar wrap.
Dinner: turkey taco lettuce wraps.

Conclusion

So, how do you feel about the ketogenic diet, now?

At first, the ketogenic diet may seem a little complicated and it may be scary, but once you get the right explanation and you have a chance to really see what kind of food you eat, you'll realize that the keto diet is one that is quite sustainable. Many people are afraid of diets for the sole reason of being afraid of getting hungry; that is one thing that you will never have to worry about with the keto diet.

As you can see from the meal plan laid out in the past few pages, the last thing you will feel is hungry. You will become healthier, energized, and lose weight. Pair this with some light exercise and you will have the toned, healthy body that you've been dreaming of.

Resources

https://ketodietapp.com/Blog/post/2013/11/05/Types-of-Ketogenic-Diets-and-the-KetoDiet-Approach

https://www.bodybuilding.com/content/cyclical-ketogenic-diet.html

https://www.ruled.me/guide-keto-diet/

http://www.mayoclinic.org/diseases-conditions/metabolic-syndrome/home/ovc-20197517

https://www.alexfergus.com/blog/24-benefits-of-the-ketogenic-diet

https://www.alexfergus.com/blog/24-benefits-of-the-ketogenic-diet

http://www.superskinnyme.com/body-measurements.html

http://dietmdhawaii.com/prescription-weight-loss/consult-your-doctor-before-weight-loss/

http://www.nhs.uk/chq/Pages/how-can-i-work-out-my-bmi.aspx?CategoryID=51

https://paleomagazine.com/what-is-keto-flu-how-to-cure-keto-flu

https://authoritynutrition.com/good-carbs-bad-carbs/

https://www.theguardian.com/lifeandstyle/2014/aug/05/where-buy-safer-healthier-more-sustainable-meat-chicken

http://www.doe.in.gov/sites/default/files/nutrition/criteria-guides.pdf

http://www.webmd.com/diet/obesity/features/skinny-fat-good-fats-bad-fats#1

http://www.eatthis.com/healthy-fats

https://www.google.ca/search?q=above+ground+vegetables&rlz=1C5CHFA_enCA742CA742&source=lnms&tbm=isch&sa=X&ved=0ahUKEwiw-IqaurHVAhUF04MKHanDBO8Q_AUICigB&biw=718&bih=803#imgrc=iyeKvQAAL-YvfM:

https://www.ruled.me/ketogenic-diet-food-list/

http://www.healthline.com/health/best-low-sugar-fruits#3

http://www.healthline.com/health/food-nutrition/greek-yogurt-benefits#protein3

https://www.dietdoctor.com/recipes/cheese-omelet

https://www.dietdoctor.com/recipes/no-bread-breakfast-sandwich

https://www.dietdoctor.com/recipes/egg-butter-smoked-salmon-avocado

https://www.dietdoctor.com/recipes/egg-muffins

https://www.tasteaholics.com/recipes/breakfast-recipes/chicken-and-zucchini-breakfast-quiche/

https://www.grassfedgirl.com/chicken-broccoli-casserole/

http://thestayathomechef.com/healthy-tuna-stuffed-avocado/#_a5y_p=3596292

http://joyfilledeats.com/bbq-bacon-cheddar-meatloaf/

https://www.thatslowcarb.com/low-carb-keto-blt-salad-recipe/#_a5y_p=6127884

http://www.cookingclassy.com/turkey-taco-lettuce-wraps/

https://www.ruled.me/salmon-patties-fresh-herbs/

https://www.essentialketo.com/easy-keto-lunches-for-work/

http://www.lecremedelacrumb.com/easy-healthy-baked-lemon-chicken/

https://www.beachbodyondemand.com/blog/cauliflower-bread-recipe

https://www.tasteofhome.com/recipes/homemade-turkey-soup

Printed in Great Britain
by Amazon